TESTICULAR CANCER ALERT

Know More About The Causes Symptoms And Treatments Of Testicular Cancer

By

Mary J. Douglas

TABLE OF CONTENTS

INTRODUCTION

The male reproductive organ known as the testicles, which are found in the scrotum, can develop cancer. This type of cancer is known as testicular cancer. Although it makes up just 1% of all male cancers, testicular cancer is the most prevalent disease in young men between the ages of 15 and 35.

A painless lump or enlargement in one of the testicles is typically the first sign of testicular cancer, which may also be followed by a heaviness or dull aching in the scrotum. A change in the testicle's size or form, a sensation of warmth or discomfort in the afflicted area, or a perception of fluid collection in the scrotum.

Although the specific etiology of testicular cancer is unknown, certain risk factors, such as a family history of the disease, an undescended testicle, or a history of testicular cancer in the other testicle, may enhance a person's chance of getting it.

Surgery to remove the damaged testis is usually followed by chemotherapy or radiation therapy to eradicate any leftover cancer cells in testicular cancer patients. The prognosis for testicular cancer is often positive, with a high likelihood of cure, provided it's discovered and treated early.

Those at risk for testicular cancer include the following:

- Age: Men between the ages of 15 and 35 are most likely to get testicular cancer.
- Race and ethnicity: White males are more likely than men of other races and ethnicities to acquire testicular cancer.
- Family history: Men who have a history of testicular cancer in their family are more likely to get the illness.
- Genetics: Klinefelter syndrome is one genetic disorder that has been linked to an increased risk of testicular cancer.
- A testicle that did not descend into the scrotum during development increases a man's risk of developing testicular cancer.
- Testicular trauma: Men who have experienced testicular trauma or injury may be more likely to acquire testicular cancer.

The presence of one or more risk factors does not guarantee the development of testicular cancer, in fact, some men who get the disease have no recognized risk factors.

Because it can increase the likelihood of effective treatment and cure, early detection of testicular cancer is crucial. Early detection of testicular cancer usually results in smaller, less advanced tumors that are simpler to be surgically removed. Early detection may also lessen the need for more severe therapies like radiation or chemotherapy, which can have serious adverse effects. Men are advised to do regular self-examinations and to visit a doctor if they find any changes or anomalies in their testicles. Additionally, it's crucial to visit the doctor for routine examinations and tests, particularly if you have testicular cancer risk factors. Regular medical checkups and self-examination can aid in early detection and treatment.

Chapter 1

Understanding Testicular Cancer

The Anatomy and Functions of the Testicles

The male reproductive system includes oval-shaped glands called testis, sometimes known as testicles. They are found inside the scrotum, a skin-covered pouch that hangs loosely from the penis. Sperm and the male sex hormone testosterone are created in the testicles and are required for reproduction.

The tunica albuginea, a thick, fibrous coat that covers the testicles, helps to shield them from harm. Sperm are created inside the testicles in a procedure known as spermatogenesis in microscopic tubes called seminiferous tubules. Before being expelled during ejaculation, the sperm first pass via several ducts, including the epididymis and vas deferens.

The development of male secondary sexual traits, such as facial hair, a deeper voice, and muscle growth, is caused by testosterone, which is also produced by the testicles in addition to sperm. In addition, testosterone contributes to the preservation of muscle mass, bone density, and red blood cell synthesis.

Overall, the testicles, which are in charge of producing both sperm and testosterone, are an essential component of the male reproductive system. Maintaining reproductive health and spotting possible problems like testicular cancer, you need knowledge of the anatomy and functions of the testicles.

Types and Stages of Testicular Cancer.

Testicular cancer can come in two primary forms, namely seminoma and non-seminoma.

- **Seminoma testicular cancer**

Testicular cancer that develops from the cells that make sperm is known as seminoma testicular cancer. It usually has a modest growth rate and responds to radiation treatment rather than chemotherapy. Seminomas are less common in elderly men and more common in males in their 30s and 40s.

Seminomas are often identified using a combination of physical examination, laboratory tests, and imaging studies like ultrasound or CT scans. The most common form of treatment for seminoma testicular cancer is radical inguinal orchiectomy, which entails surgically removing the afflicted testicle. Depending on the cancer's stage and extent, extra treatment may be required after surgery. Chemotherapy, radiation therapy, or a combination of the two might be used in this situation.

Seminoma testicular cancer has an excellent prognosis, and early-stage seminomas have a cure rate of above 95%. To watch for any indications of recurrence or the development of new cancers, it is crucial to schedule routine follow-up sessions with a healthcare professional.

- **Non-seminoma testicular cancer**

Testicular cancer of the non-seminoma variety develops in the cells of the testicles. Teratoma, yolk sac carcinoma, embryonal carcinoma, and choriocarcinoma are the four most prevalent kinds of non-seminoma testicular cancer. These tumors need more intensive therapy because they often spread more quickly than seminoma testicular cancers. A tumor or lump in one of the testicles is the most typical sign of non-seminoma testicular cancer. A dull aching in the lower abdomen, a rapid buildup of fluid in the scrotum, and an enlargement or tenderness of the breasts are a few additional symptoms that could be present.

Surgery to remove the malignant testicle, chemotherapy, radiation therapy, or a combination of these treatments are frequently used as treatments for non-seminoma testicular cancer. Treatment aims to eradicate the cancer and stop it from spreading to other bodily regions.

It is significant to remember that non-seminoma testicular cancer, when discovered early, is very curable. You should schedule an appointment with your doctor right away to get checked if you experience any of the symptoms of non-seminoma testicular cancer.

Testicular cancer Stages

The process of estimating the degree or severity of cancer in the body is referred to as cancer staging. Staging aids medical professionals in selecting the best course of action and prognosis for each patient. The size of the tumor, whether it has progressed to neighboring lymph nodes or other organs, and if it has metastasized (spread) to distant regions of the body are all considered when determining the stage of cancer.

Stage 1

The initial stage of the disease, stage 1 testicular cancer, indicates that the cancer is contained to the testis and has not migrated to adjacent lymph nodes or other body organs. Stage 1 testicular cancer is typically curable with surgery alone, without the use of other therapies like chemotherapy or radiation.

A radical inguinal orchiectomy, which involves the surgical removal of the afflicted testis, is the conventional course of treatment for stage 1 testicular cancer. This technique is usually carried out as an outpatient surgery, is low-risk, and has few consequences. After surgery, it's crucial to schedule routine follow-up visits with a healthcare professional to check for any indications of recurrence or the development of new cancers.

For stage 1 testicular cancer, extra therapy may occasionally be advised, especially if certain risk factors are present, such as big tumor size or invasion of blood arteries or lymphatic systems. Radiation therapy and chemotherapy are potential further therapies, though these are typically saved for situations when there is a high chance of recurrence.

With a cure rate of more than 99%, stage 1 testicular cancer has an outstanding overall prognosis. To watch for any indications of recurrence or the development of new cancers, it is crucial to schedule routine follow-up sessions with a healthcare professional.

Stage 2

The liver or lungs are among the distal lymph nodes or organs where the malignancy has spread. Testicular cancer in stage 2 has spread to adjacent lymph nodes in addition to the testis but has not yet reached other body organs. Chemotherapy and surgery are frequently used in conjunction as a kind of treatment for stage 2 testicular cancer.

A radical inguinal orchiectomy to remove the afflicted testis is typically the first line of treatment for stage 2 testicular cancer. After surgery, further therapy could be required to get rid of any cancer cells that remained. Chemotherapy, radiation treatment, or a combination of the two may be used in this situation. Depending on the subtype of testicular cancer and the degree of disease metastasis, a particular chemotherapy regimen may be utilised. If the cancer is chemotherapy-resistant, radiation therapy may also be utilised to target particular parts of the body where the disease has spread.

Stage 2 testicular cancer has a favourable prognosis and a cure rate of over 90%. To watch for any indications of recurrence or the development of new cancers, schedule routine follow-up sessions with your healthcare professional. It is significant to highlight that fertility and sexual function may be impacted by testicular cancer treatment. Before starting therapy, men who are worried about their fertility or sexual performance should talk to their doctor about their concerns.

Stage 3

The most advanced stage of testicular cancer is stage 3, which denotes that the illness has spread to the lymph nodes, lungs, liver, or brain in addition to the testicle. Additionally, the cancer may have migrated to distant organs like the abdomen or bones.

The following are examples of stage 3 testicular cancer symptoms:

- Neck, armpit, or groin lymph node swelling or tumors
- Breathing problems or shortness of breath
- Chest pains
- Blood in the cough

- Pain or edema in the abdomen
- Vomiting or nauseous
- Migraines or seizures
- Fractures or pain in the bones

Imaging techniques, such as CT scans, MRIs, or PET scans, which can identify the presence and location of malignant cells in the body, are frequently used to diagnose stage 3 testicular cancer. The existence and extent of testicular cancer can be determined by blood tests that check the levels of tumor markers such as alpha-fetoprotein (AFP), beta-human chorionic gonadotropin (beta-hCG), and lactate dehydrogenase (LDH).

Depending on the location and severity of the tumour, a combination of surgery, chemotherapy, and radiation therapy is frequently used to treat stage 3 testicular cancer. The afflicted testicle and any neighbouring lymph nodes may be surgically removed, and chemotherapy and radiation therapy may be utilised to eradicate any cancer cells that have metastasized to other body organs. The proliferation of hormone-sensitive testicular cancer cells can also be slowed down by hormone therapy.

The prognosis for stage 3 testicular cancer relies on many variables, including the disease's kind and stage, the patient's age and general health, and how well they respond to treatment. The five-year survival rate for stage 3 testicular cancer is approximately 73%, however, it is normally good with early discovery and the right treatment.

With a five-year survival rate of over 95% for all stages combined, testicular cancer is typically regarded as a relatively treatable kind of cancer. To get the best results, though, early detection and timely treatment are essential.

Signs and Symptoms of Testicular Cancer

A painless lump or enlargement in one or both testicles is frequently the first sign of testicular cancer. There may also be additional indicators of testicular cancer, such as:

- Lower abdominal or scrotal pain that feels heavy or oraches.
- Scrotal or testicular pain or discomfort.
- Testicle or scrotum swelling or lumps.
- Gynecomastia, an enlargement or discomfort of the breast tissue.
- Backache.
- Pain or swelling in the abdomen.
- Weakness or exhaustion.
- Unexpected weight loss.

It is crucial to remember that some of these symptoms could also be brought on by other health issues, such as an infection, damage, or non-cancerous growth in the testicles. However, it's crucial to contact a doctor for an assessment and accurate diagnosis if you have any of these symptoms.

Chapter 2

Diagnosis and Testing

Self-Examination

Testicular self-examination is an important element of preserving male reproductive health. It is recommended that men undertake a self-examination once a month to look for any abnormalities or changes in the testicles.

Here are the steps for completing a testicular self-examination:

- Start by standing in front of a mirror and visually evaluating the scrotum for any edema or anomalies.

- Next, carefully feel each testicle with both hands, using your fingers and thumb to roll the testicle between them. You should feel for any lumps, bumps, or changes in size or shape.

- Repeat the process with the other testicle.

- Finally, inspect the epididymis, which is a tiny, tube-like structure located at the back of each testicle. It should feel soft and smooth, and any lumps or bumps should be reported to a doctor.

It is crucial to note that not all lumps or bumps in the testicles are malignant, but any changes should be evaluated by a doctor. Testicular cancer is rare but can be quite aggressive, therefore early discovery is important for successful treatment.

If you observe any changes during self-examination or have any worries about your testicular health, it is crucial to schedule an appointment with a doctor or urologist as soon as possible.

Medical Examination And Imaging Tests

If a doctor suspects that a man may have testicular cancer, they may offer a set of tests to diagnose the illness. These tests may include:

- **Physical exam:** The doctor will examine the testicles, scrotum, groin, and abdomen for any abnormalities, tumours, or swelling.
- **Blood tests:** Blood tests can be done to check for tumour markers, which are chemicals produced by some types of cancer cells. In regards to testicular cancer, the tumour marker is most often alpha-

fetoprotein (AFP) or human chorionic gonadotropin (HCG).

- **Ultrasound:** An ultrasound employs high-frequency sound waves to obtain images of the interior anatomy of the testicles. This test can help detect if a lump is solid or fluid-filled and can help identify if it is likely to be malignant or not.

Biopsy and Pathology Reports

Biopsy

A biopsy is a medical operation in which a small sample of tissue is taken from the body for examination under a microscope. In the instance of testicular cancer, a biopsy may be conducted to confirm the presence of malignant cells.

The biopsy technique for testicular cancer is usually done under local anaesthetic, and the sample is extracted through a small incision in the scrotum. The tissue sample is subsequently delivered to a laboratory for analysis by a pathologist.

The pathologist will analyse the tissue sample under a microscope and look for the presence of abnormal cells. They will also assess the type and stage of the cancer, which will help select the best course of therapy.

The pathology report will include information regarding the type of cancer cells present, including the degree of differentiation or how much the cancer cells resemble normal testicular cells. The report will also include information regarding the stage of cancer, which is determined by the size of the tumor and if it has spread to other parts of the body.

Pathology report

This is a crucial tool for doctors in evaluating the best therapy options for the patient. Options for treatment may include surgery, radiation therapy, chemotherapy, or a combination of these treatments. It is crucial to realise that not all testicular tumours or anomalies are malignant, and many are benign. However, any odd symptoms or changes in the testicles should be evaluated by a specialist, and a biopsy may be needed to rule out malignancy.

Chapter 3

Options for Treatment

Surgery

Orchiectomy

One or both testicles may be removed through a surgical operation called an orchiectomy. It is a typical treatment for testicular cancer and can either be used to diagnose the disease or treat it.

Orchiectomy may be suggested as the initial course of treatment if a biopsy reveals the existence of testicular cancer. Through a groin incision, the diseased testicle is removed during the surgery.

The excised testicle is submitted to a lab for analysis after the operation to confirm the diagnosis and establish the kind and stage of cancer. Additional therapies, such as chemotherapy, may be used if the cancer is discovered to be more advanced or to have spread to other parts of the body.

It is crucial to remember that losing one testicle typically has no impact on a man's ability to have intercourse or produce children. Frequently, the surviving testicle can produce enough testosterone and sperm to preserve fertility and normal sexual function.

Even though it may seem like a severe measure, an orchiectomy is frequently required as part of the treatment of testicular cancer. Most men can resume their normal activities after a few weeks of the surgery, and the technique has a high success rate.

Retroperitoneal Lymph Node Dissection

Dissection of the retroperitoneal lymph nodes testicular cancer treatment occasionally includes a surgical technique known as retroperitoneal lymph node dissection (RPLND).

The treatment normally necessitates a few days in the hospital and is performed under general anaesthesia. The surgeon will make an incision in the belly and take the lymph nodes out of the retroperitoneal region during the procedure. Depending on the cancer's stage and location, the degree of the lymph node ectomy will vary.

In circumstances when the cancer has gone to the lymph nodes, RPLND can be a successful treatment for testicular cancer. However, there are certain potential dangers and consequences associated with the treatment, including bleeding, infection, and harm to surrounding organs or nerves.

Patients will typically need to stay in the hospital for a few days following the procedure, and they will need to adhere to a rehabilitation schedule that includes rest, medication, monitoring the pains, and keeping an eye out for any potential problems. To track the patient's progress and make sure the malignancy has been successfully treated, follow-up care will also be required.

Overall, RPLND may have a significant role in the management of testicular cancer, especially when the disease has progressed to the lymph nodes. However, the choice to have the surgery should be made in collaboration with a doctor, who will also consider the patient's general health and the procedure's advantages and disadvantages.

Chemotherapy

Chemotherapy is frequently used to treat testicular cancer, particularly when the disease has progressed to other body organs. Chemotherapy, which can be administered orally or intravenously, uses chemicals to kill cancer cells.

Cisplatin, etoposide, and bleomycin are frequently combined as medications used in chemotherapy for testicular cancer. The kind, stage, and length of the cancer, as well as the patient's general health, will determine the precise chemotherapy regimen and duration.

Chemotherapy for testicular cancer is typically administered in cycles, with a treatment phase followed by a recovery phase. Depending on the cancer's severity and the patient's reaction to the treatment, the treatment cycle can last anywhere from a few weeks to a few months.

Chemotherapy has negative effects even if it can be a successful treatment for testicular cancer and frequently causes side effects including nausea, vomiting, exhaustion, hair loss, and an increased risk of infection. However, the majority of negative effects, nevertheless, can be controlled with medicine or other therapies.

Patients will require routine follow-up appointments and monitoring following chemotherapy to make sure the cancer has been successfully treated. If the cancer comes back or if any cancer cells remain in some circumstances, more therapies can be required.

In general, chemotherapy can play a significant role in the management of testicular cancer, especially when the disease has gone beyond the testicles. However, the choice to receive chemotherapy should be taken after seeing a doctor and taking into account the patient's general health as well as the risks and advantages of the procedure.

The majority of negative effects, nevertheless, can be controlled with medicine or other therapies.

Types, Adverse Effects, And Administration

Combinations of medications that are given intravenously or orally are the most popular types of chemotherapy used to treat testicular cancer. The kind and stage of cancer determine the precise medications used and the length of the course of treatment. The most typical chemotherapy plans for testicular cancer are as follows:

BEP: This treatment plan contains the medications cisplatin, bleomycin, and etoposide. It is used to treat testicular cancer at all stages and is the most popular chemotherapy treatment. The acronym BEP refers to a chemotherapy treatment plan frequently used to treat testicular cancer that has spread beyond the testicles. It is typical to provide this medication in cycles, with each cycle lasting roughly three weeks. Depending on the unique circumstances and the patient's response to treatment, the number of cycles and dosage of the medications employed may change. Although testicular cancer has been demonstrated to respond very well to BEP treatment, there are some possible side effects, including nausea, hair loss, and an elevated risk of infection. Before starting BEP medication, it's crucial to go over the potential risks and advantages with a doctor.

EP: This medication combination includes cisplatin and etoposide. It is frequently used as an alternative to the BEP regimen and is used to treat testicular cancer that is in the early stages. A frequent form of treatment for testicular cancer is EP chemotherapy. This stops the cells from proliferating and dividing, which ultimately causes them to die.

Another chemotherapy medication that affects cancer cells' DNA is called cisplatin. Additionally, this stops the cells from growing and dividing, which causes them to die.

A potent chemotherapy regimen that can successfully target and eliminate cancer cells in the testicles is made up of the drugs etoposide and cisplatin when used together.

EP chemotherapy is frequently administered in cycles, each of which lasts roughly three weeks. The patient will be given both medications intravenously (via an IV) at a medical facility during this period.

EP chemotherapy side effects can include diarrhoea, vomiting, hair loss, exhaustion, and a compromised immune system. However, most individuals can manage these adverse effects with medication and lifestyle adjustments and the majority of patients can finish their treatment without experiencing serious consequences.

It's vital to remember that not every patient with testicular cancer should have EP chemotherapy. The type and stage of the patient's cancer, as well as other personal circumstances, can affect the treatment options. As a result, patients must consult with their medical professionals frequently to develop the optimal treatment strategy for their circumstances.

VIP: In this treatment plan, cisplatin, etoposide, and ifosfamide are all taken together if the BEP regimen is ineffective. It is frequently used to treat testicular cancer that has progressed to that stage. By inhibiting DNA replication and harming cancer cells' DNA, respectively, etoposide and cisplatin operate similarly to how they do in EP chemotherapy. Ifosfamide, a chemotherapy medication, operates differently and prevents the cell from being able to divide and expand.

VIP chemotherapy is likewise administered in cycles, which normally last three weeks. The patient will be given intravenously (via an IV) at a medical facility all three medications during this period.

Similar to EP chemotherapy, VIP chemotherapy can also have negative side effects such as nausea, vomiting, hair loss, exhaustion, and a compromised immune system. The particular side effects and their intensity, however, can change depending on the patient as a whole and their general health.

As with any cancer treatment, patients should consult closely with their medical professionals to choose the course of action that will work best for them. For some patients with testicular cancer, VIP chemotherapy may not be the best option; instead, surgery or radiation therapy may be a better course of action.

4. **TIP:** Another approach for treating testicular cancer is TIP chemotherapy. It consists of the medicines paclitaxel, ifosfamide, and cisplatin in combination.

A chemotherapy medicine called paclitaxel inhibits cancer cells' ability to divide through cell division. This stops the cells from expanding and finally causes them to die. Similar to how they do in VIP chemotherapy, ifosfamide and cisplatin affect cancer cells' DNA and interfere with cell division, respectively.

TIP chemotherapy is frequently administered in cycles, each of which lasts for roughly three weeks. The patient will be given intravenously (via an IV) at a medical facility all three medications during this period.

TIP chemotherapy, like other chemotherapies, can have negative side effects including nausea, vomiting, hair loss, exhaustion, and a compromised immune system.

The particular side effects and their intensity, however, can change depending on the patient as a whole and their general health.

TIP chemotherapy is frequently used as a salvage therapy for patients whose testicular cancer has returned or progressed following the first therapy. Patients who have advanced or metastatic testicular cancer can also receive it as their initial line of treatment.

As with any cancer treatment, patients should consult closely with their medical professionals to choose the course of action that will work best for them. TIP Other forms of treatment, such as surgery or radiation therapy, may be more suitable for certain patients with testicular cancer than chemotherapy. The type and stage of cancer, as well as the patient's general health and treatment response, all influence the choice of chemotherapy plan. A doctor will decide the precise medications to be used and the length of the treatment after thoroughly assessing the patient's health.

Radiation Therapy

Although it is less frequently used than chemotherapy, radiation therapy is another option for treating testicular cancer. To eradicate cancer cells, high-energy radiation is used to kill the cancer cells in the testicles Depending on the type and stage of cancer as well as the patient's general condition, radiation therapy may be administered alone or in conjunction with chemotherapy.

The patient receives high-energy radiation while they receive radiation therapy while they are lying on a table. The procedure is normally administered over weeks in daily sessions.

Fatigue, skin irritation or dryness in the treated area, nausea, and diarrhoea are possible side effects of radiation therapy. These side effects can be treated with medicine and dietary adjustments, however, they are frequently transient.

Given that radiation therapy has been demonstrated to be extremely effective in treating stage I seminoma testicular cancer, it may be suggested for patients with this condition.

Patients with stage II or stage III seminoma or non-seminoma testicular cancer may also be treated with it, while chemotherapy is frequently the recommended course of action in these circumstances. As with any cancer treatment, patients should consult closely with their medical professionals to choose the course of action that will work best for them. For certain patients with testicular cancer, radiation therapy may not be the best course of action; instead, chemotherapy or surgery may be preferable.

Techniques of Radiation Therapy

Depending on the stage and location of the disease as well as the patient's general condition, a variety of radiation treatment procedures may be utilised to treat testicular cancer. These methods consist of:

External beam radiation

This is the most popular form of radiation therapy for treating testicular cancer. It involves delivering high-energy radiation to the damaged area from outside the body using a device known as a linear accelerator. The testicles and adjacent lymph nodes are the intended targets of the radiation.

Brachytherapy: This form of radiation treatment involves injecting minute radioactive seeds or pellets into the body, either directly into the afflicted area or close by. This reduces radiation exposure to healthy tissues while still delivering a high dose of radiation directly to the cancer cells.

Proton therapy: This type of radiation treatment targets cancer cells with high-energy protons rather than X-rays. Although it is less common than other radiation therapies, it may be utilised in select cases of testicular cancer.

Intensity-modulated radiation treatment (IMRT): This external beam radiation therapy employs cutting-edge computer software to give extremely accurate radiation dosages to the affected area. This minimises radiation exposure to healthy tissues while delivering a higher dose of radiation to the cancer cells.

Stereotactic body radiation therapy (SBRT): Compared to conventional radiation therapy, SBRT combines cutting-edge imaging technology to give very precise radiation doses to the afflicted area in fewer treatments. Some cases of testicular cancer that have progressed to the neighborhood lymph nodes might be treated with it.

As with any cancer treatment, patients should consult closely with their medical professionals to choose the course of action that will work best for them. For certain patients with testicular cancer, radiation therapy may not be the best course of action; instead, chemotherapy or surgery may be preferable.

Risks

Testicular cancer is frequently treated with radiation therapy, but like all medical interventions, there are potential side effects. Radiation therapy for testicular cancer carries some hazards, such as:

- **Healthy tissue damage:** Radiation therapy has the potential to harm healthy tissue close to the testicles, which may result in side effects like exhaustion, skin rashes, and hair loss.
- **Infertility:** Radiation treatment can harm the testicles and lower sperm production, which might cause infertility.
- **Subsequent cancers:** Although the risk is often modest, radiation therapy can raise the chance of the later-life development of second cancer.
- **Hormonal changes:** Radiation therapy may alter how the body produces hormones, which may result in symptoms including erectile dysfunction, heat flashes, and diminished sex drive.
- **Long-term adverse effects:** Some radiation therapy side effects, like infertility

and hormone abnormalities, might last a lifetime.

It's critical to remember that radiation therapy hazards differ based on the patient and the particular treatment plan. Before you start radiation therapy, your doctor will go through all of the possible risks and advantages with you in great detail.

Chapter Four

Coping with Testicular Cancer

Psychological and Emotional Effects

A person may experience substantial emotional and psychological effects after receiving a testicular cancer diagnosis. Following a testicular cancer diagnosis, frequently emotional and psychological reactions include the following:

- **Shock and disbelief:** Learning that you have cancer can be devastating, and it's not uncommon for people to feel surprised, numb, and overwhelmed.

- **Dread and anxiety:** Feelings of dread and anxiety might be brought on by the uncertainty of cancer therapy and the potential for recurrence.

- **Depression:** Many cancer patients develop depressive symptoms including melancholy, hopelessness, and losing interest in once-enjoyed activities.

- **Anger and frustration:** Cancer patients frequently experience anger or frustration over their diagnosis, course of treatment, or how cancer has affected their lives.

- **Body image issues:** The removal of one or both testicles as part of testicular cancer therapy can occasionally cause body image issues as well as feelings of inferiority or emasculation.

- **Relationship difficulties:** In addition to affecting sexual intimacy and fertility, cancer can cause problems in relationships with partners, family members, and friends.

- **Money issues:** Cancer treatment can be costly, and the financial strain can exacerbate the stress and anxiety that come with receiving a cancer diagnosis.

When dealing with the difficulties of cancer therapy and trying to enhance their quality of life, patients with testicular cancer should seek out emotional and psychological support. This could entail finding alternative sources of emotional support, speaking with a therapist or counsellor, joining a support group, etc.

Speaking with Family and Friends

It might be challenging to inform family and friends that you have testicular cancer, but it's crucial to have their support during this tough time. Here are some pointers for explaining your diagnosis to your loved ones:

- **Pick the correct time and location**

Select a time and location where you feel relaxed and have privacy to speak. Do not discuss your diagnosis in front of others or when you are stressed out.

- **Be upfront and honest**

It's crucial to be open and honest about your diagnosis, treatment strategy, and emotional state. Discuss with your family and friends how they can be of help to you.

- **Provide details**

Disclose details on testicular cancer, its treatment, and what to anticipate. Your loved ones will be better able to support you if they know what you are going through.

- **Communicate your emotions**

Whether you're afraid, angry, or sad, it's normal to communicate your sentiments. Even if they might be at a loss for words, your loved ones can still listen and be supportive.

- **Don't be hesitant to seek assistance**

This goes for both practical and emotional support. Your loved ones might want to encourage you but are unsure of how to do so.

- **Have patience**

Allow your loved ones some time to take in the information and adjust to the circumstances. They might need to process their own emotions and sensations.

There is no right or wrong way to feel or respond to cancer; just keep in mind that everyone deals with it in their unique way. If you require more assistance dealing with your illness and communicating with your loved ones, look for assistance from a therapist, counsellor.

Support Resources and Survivorship Care

For those who have testicular cancer, support systems, and survivorship care are crucial.

The following are some of the potential resources and services:

- **Support groups**

Becoming a member of a support group can offer mental and emotional assistance as well as a sense of belonging. Support groups can be run by peers or healthcare professionals and can take place offline or online.

- **Counselling**

Speaking with a therapist or counsellor can assist you in coping with the emotional and psychological effects of cancer.

- **Survivorship care plans**

These individualised plans offer details on post-treatment care, potential long-term impacts, and measures to maintain general health and wellness.

- **Rehabilitation services**

Services like physical therapy, which are part of the rehabilitation process, can assist in managing the physical side effects of cancer treatment, such as pain, weakness, and exhaustion.

- **Financial support**

Programs that can help with the cost of cancer treatment and associated costs like travel and lodging may be available.

- **Palliative care**

This is a type of specialist medical care that focuses on enhancing the quality of life for cancer patients by reducing pain and controlling symptoms.

- **Clinical trials:**

Testicular cancer patients who are interested in taking part in research studies to advance cancer treatment may be able to find clinical trials.

It's vital to discuss the resources and services that are available to you with your healthcare team. They can direct you to local support groups, set you up with a therapist or counsellor, and provide you with details about survivorship care plans and other tools.

Chapter 5

Healthy Living with Testicular Cancer

Dietary and exercise recommendations

Exercise and proper nutrition are crucial for overall health and well-being, but they can be even more crucial for those who have testicular cancer. Here are some general recommendations for diet and activity for those with testicular cancer:

Nutrition:

- Consume an array of fruits, vegetables, whole grains, lean meats, and healthy fats as part of a balanced diet. This can help you keep a healthy weight while giving your body the nutrition it requires for recuperation and restoration.
- Maintain adequate hydration: Drinking plenty of liquids, particularly water, will help prevent dehydration and enhance general health.

- Keep alcohol and caffeine intake to a minimum. These substances can disrupt sleep and may make certain cancer treatment side effects worse.
- Think about collaborating with a trained dietitian: A registered dietitian may assist you in developing a personalised nutrition strategy that takes into account your unique requirements and preferences.

Exercise:

- Consult with your healthcare team before beginning an exercise regimen to ensure that it is safe for you and to get suggestions for the kind and level of exercise that is right for you.
- Start slowly: It's crucial to start slowly and gradually increase the intensity and duration of your workout program if you haven't been active in a while.
- Select low-impact exercises: Low-impact exercises can be easier on your muscles and joints and may be a good place to start. Examples include walking, swimming, and cycling.

- Include weightlifting: Weightlifting can help maintain muscle mass and enhance bone density, both of which can be crucial for overall health.
- Pay attention to your body: It's critical to pay attention to your body and avoid overexerting yourself. Rest as necessary, and don't be afraid to ask for assistance or change your exercise regimen if you're in pain or uncomfortable.

Every person has different demands and restrictions, so it's important to collaborate with your healthcare team to develop a nutrition and fitness plan that is suited to your particular requirements.

Sexual Health and Fertility Concerns

Men's fertility and sexual health may be impacted by testicular cancer and its treatment. Here are a few typical issues and suggestions for sexual and reproductive health

- **Erectile dysfunction**

Chemotherapy, radiation therapy, and surgery can all lead to erectile dysfunction (ED). ED can be treated with drugs like sildenafil (Viagra), tadalafil (Cialis), or vardenafil (Levitra).

- **Libido loss**

Both testicular cancer and its treatment can reduce a person's desire for sex. Managing side effects and discussing treatment options with a healthcare professional can help libido.

- **Concerns about fertility**

Testicular cancer and its treatment may have an impact on fertility. Before therapy, sperm banking or cryopreservation can protect a patient's capacity to have biological children in the future.

- **Hormonal imbalances**

Some testicular cancer treatments have the potential to alter hormone levels, which can result in symptoms including hot flashes, exhaustion, and a decline in libido. The use of hormone replacement therapy could be beneficial.

- **Body image issues**

Testicular cancer therapy, like surgery to remove a testis, can affect one's self-esteem and body image.

These issues may be addressed by therapy or counselling.

- **Communication with partners**

Sexual relationships and communication with partners may be impacted by testicular cancer and its treatment. To maintain intimacy and resolve concerns, communication that is open and honest is crucial.

Discussing sexual and reproductive health issues with healthcare professionals is vital because they can advise on available treatments and make referrals to experts like urologists or reproductive endocrinologists. Before beginning therapy, sperm banking should be addressed with a doctor because the procedure can take many weeks to complete.

Follow-Up Care and Monitoring

Follow-up care and surveillance are crucial after treatment for testicular cancer to spot any potential recurrence or long-lasting effects of the medication. Here are some general recommendations for monitoring and follow-up care:

- Regular physical examinations can assist identify any changes or abnormalities, including testicular examinations.

-

- Blood testing, like tumour marker tests, can assist identify any indications of a cancer recurrence.

-

- Imaging studies: To check for any indications of a cancer recurrence, imaging tests like CT scans or X-rays may be advised.

- Testicular self-examinations can assist in identifying any alterations or anomalies in the testicles.

- Survivorship care plans: These plans offer details on how to maintain general health and wellness, probable long-term impacts of therapy, and follow-up care.

- Lifestyle changes: Changing one's habits, such as giving up smoking, eating healthily, and exercising frequently, can enhance general well-being and lower the risk of cancer recurrence.

An individual's particular cancer diagnosis and treatment plan will determine the type, frequency, and follow-up care and monitoring that is required. It's crucial to talk about monitoring and follow-up treatment with a healthcare professional who can provide tailored suggestions based on each patient's needs and concerns.

CONCLUSION

It is possible to survive testicular cancer, and it all begins with a good outlook and a desire to take charge of your health. One of the most treatable types of cancer, testicular cancer has a high survival rate, especially when detected early. The road to rehabilitation can be difficult, though, both physically and mentally. The following advice can help you survive testicular cancer:

- Keep up with your follow-up appointments: It's crucial to schedule regular checkups with your doctor after treatment. These visits will aid in tracking your development and identifying any signs of cancer that might come back.

- Take good care of your physical health by working out, eating well, and getting enough sleep. These lifestyle choices can help you maintain a healthy physique and lower your risk of developing additional health issues.
- Seek assistance: If you're experiencing emotional difficulty, join a cancer support group or speak with a therapist. Having an unwavering support group is very important at this time.
- Embrace life: Pay attention to the things that make you happy. Find ways to have fun and make the most of each day, whether it is by travelling, engaging in a hobby, or spending time with loved ones.
- Speak out for your health: If you have worries about your health, act as your advocate. Never hesitate to ask questions or, if necessary, seek a second opinion.
-

Keep in mind that testicular cancer can be beaten. You can prosper and have a fulfilling life if you have the appropriate perspective and assistance.

Throughout history, humans have shown an incredible ability to adapt and overcome even the most difficult challenges. We have faced pandemics, wars, and natural disasters, but we always find a way to persevere. This resilience gives us hope that we can overcome any obstacle that comes our way.

There is hope for the future! Despite the numerous difficulties our society faces, there are numerous causes for optimism about the future.

Technology is advancing quickly and can help with many of the world's most pressing issues. Our lives are being made better by technology in various ways, from healthcare to renewable energy.

In conclusion, there is cause for hope even if there will undoubtedly be obstacles in the future. We can build a brighter future for ourselves and future generations by cooperating and remaining upbeat.